Holistic Healing: Natural Remedies for Alleviating Joint Pain

Discover Effective and Gentle Approaches to Relieve Joint Discomfort Without Pharmaceuticals

Emily Clark

Introduction

The journey to alleviating joint pain begins with an exploration of natural remedies that prioritize holistic well-being. In this guide, we delve into the intricacies of joint pain, emphasizing the significance of opting for gentle and effective solutions over conventional pharmaceuticals. By understanding the root causes and embracing lifestyle adjustments, herbal therapies, essential oils, mind-body practices, supplements, and home remedies, you'll embark on a path that not only relieves joint discomfort but also fosters overall health. Join us as we navigate the realms of natural healing to empower you on your quest for joint wellness.

In this exploration of natural remedies for joint pain, we've unveiled a comprehensive guide that goes beyond mere relief, aiming to empower you on a transformative journey towards holistic well-being. As we delve into the intricacies of joint discomfort and the various natural avenues available for support, remember that this guide is not just about managing symptoms—it's about fostering a sustainable and balanced approach to joint care. Join us in navigating the realms of lifestyle adjustments, herbal therapies, essential oils, and more, as we embark together on a path towards not only alleviating joint pain but also enhancing your overall quality of life.

Understanding Joint Pain

we unravel the complexities of joint pain, delving into the anatomy and common causes behind discomfort. Gain insights into how factors like inflammation, aging, and lifestyle contribute to joint issues. By comprehending the intricacies of joint pain, you'll be better equipped to tailor natural remedies to address specific challenges and promote sustained relief. Let's explore the foundations of joint pain and pave the way for a more informed approach to holistic healing.

Within the complex landscape of joint pain, our exploration goes beyond surface discomfort, aiming to unravel the nuanced factors contributing to your experience. From the physiological intricacies to the impact of lifestyle, we delve into a comprehensive understanding. Recognizing joint pain as more than a symptom, this section illuminates the interplay of inflammation, aging, and daily habits. By grasping the intricacies, you are better equipped to tailor your holistic approach—addressing not just the pain, but the root causes. Join us in this deep dive into understanding joint pain for a more informed and personalized journey toward relief and resilience.

The Importance of Natural Remedies

Discover why embracing natural remedies is pivotal in the journey towards joint wellness. Uncover the advantages of opting for holistic approaches over conventional medications, exploring the gentle yet effective ways in which natural remedies can alleviate joint pain. From minimizing side effects to promoting overall health, this section highlights the inherent benefits of choosing nature's solutions for joint discomfort. Explore how a holistic mindset can contribute not only to symptom relief but also to a more balanced and sustainable approach to joint care.

In emphasizing the importance of natural remedies, we underscore a paradigm shift towards gentle, sustainable approaches in joint care. This transcends mere symptom management, advocating for a deeper connection with your body's innate healing capacities. Natural remedies offer not just relief from joint pain but a holistic enhancement of overall health. By choosing nature's pathways, you embrace solutions that often carry fewer side effects, aligning with your body's natural rhythms. This section champions the notion that, beyond addressing symptoms, natural remedies become companions in a journey toward long-term well-being, allowing you to reclaim agency over your health in a balanced and harmonious way.

Chapter 1
Lifestyle Adjustments

Embark on a transformative journey by exploring lifestyle adjustments that play a crucial role in managing and preventing joint pain. Dive into dietary modifications that support joint health and discover exercise routines and stretching techniques tailored for mobility. This section guides you in making sustainable changes to your daily life, empowering you to proactively address joint discomfort through lifestyle choices. Unlock the potential for improved joint function and overall well-being as we navigate the realm of practical and effective adjustments.

Dive deeper into the transformative potential of lifestyle adjustments, recognizing them as foundational pillars for robust joint health. From dietary shifts to exercise routines, this section guides you in cultivating habits that resonate with your body's unique needs. It's not just about adapting; it's about creating an environment conducive to joint resilience. Explore the profound impact of small, sustainable changes that ripple across your daily life, fostering not only physical well-being but a holistic sense of vitality. Join us in the exploration of lifestyle adjustments as powerful tools for crafting a life where joint health is not just a goal but an integrated and harmonious aspect of your overall wellness.

Dietary Changes for Joint Health

Discover the power of nutrition in fostering joint health. Uncover dietary changes that can positively impact inflammation and support optimal joint function. From anti-inflammatory foods to joint-friendly nutrients, this section provides practical insights and tips on how to structure a diet that promotes joint wellness.

Explore the connection between food choices and joint health, empowering yourself with the knowledge to make informed decisions for sustained comfort and mobility.

Delve into the realm of dietary changes as a key cornerstone in nurturing joint health. This section guides you through the intricacies of food choices, emphasizing the role of anti-inflammatory options and joint-friendly nutrients. Explore the profound impact of your diet on inflammation levels, cartilage health, and overall joint function. From embracing omega-3 fatty acids to incorporating antioxidants, this journey into dietary adjustments is not just about what you eat—it's about fueling your body with the elements essential for optimal joint well-being. Join us in this exploration, where your dietary choices become a proactive and delicious path to nurturing your joints.

Exercise and Stretching Routines

Unlock the potential for improved joint flexibility and strength through tailored exercise and stretching routines. Dive into exercises designed to enhance joint mobility, strengthen supporting muscles, and promote overall joint health. This section provides practical guidance on incorporating low-impact activities and targeted stretches into your routine, fostering resilience and reducing the risk of joint discomfort. Explore a holistic approach to physical well-being as we guide you through exercises that not only benefit your joints but contribute to your overall fitness and vitality.

In our exploration of exercise and stretching routines, let's delve deeper into the transformative potential of movement. Beyond the physical benefits, consider these routines as a daily ritual for nurturing joint flexibility and strength. Explore the symbiotic relationship between your muscles and joints, understanding how targeted exercises not only alleviate current discomfort but also contribute to long-term joint resilience. This section invites you to view movement not as a chore but as a mindful practice—each stretch and exercise a conscious step towards a more agile and comfortable you. Join us in unlocking the full spectrum of benefits that exercise and stretching routines offer for sustained joint health and overall well-being.

Chapter 2
Herbal Therapies

Delve into the world of herbal therapies as we explore nature's remedies for joint health. Learn about potent anti-inflammatory herbs and how they can alleviate joint discomfort. Discover the art of crafting herbal teas that not only soothe but also promote joint relief. This section unveils the diverse and time-tested herbal approaches to support your joint wellness journey. Embrace the healing power of nature as we guide you through incorporating herbal therapies into your daily routine for a holistic and gentle approach to managing joint pain.

Embark on a comprehensive exploration of herbal therapies, unraveling the rich tapestry of nature's healing potential. Beyond their role in alleviating joint pain, delve into the nuanced properties of specific herbs like turmeric, ginger, and boswellia. Understand how these botanical allies engage with your body's natural processes, providing anti-inflammatory support and promoting joint comfort. This section aims to not only introduce herbal remedies but to empower you with knowledge, enabling you to tailor your approach based on the unique characteristics of each herb. Join us in this botanical journey, where the wisdom of nature becomes a guiding force in your pursuit of holistic joint well-being.

Incorporating Anti-Inflammatory Herbs

Explore the potential of anti-inflammatory herbs in managing joint pain. Uncover the properties of herbs like turmeric, ginger, and boswellia, known for their natural anti-inflammatory effects. Learn how to incorporate these herbs into your diet and daily routine to harness their healing properties. This section provides insights into the science behind these herbs and practical tips for maximizing their benefits in promoting joint health. Discover a natural and herbal approach to combating inflammation and supporting your journey towards more comfortable and flexible joints.

In our exploration of incorporating anti-inflammatory herbs, let's deepen our understanding of their potent healing properties. Journey into the specifics of herbs like turmeric, renowned for curcumin's anti-inflammatory effects, and explore the synergy of combining these herbs for enhanced joint relief. This section guides you in crafting a personalized approach, considering factors like dosage and preparation methods. By delving into the science and artistry of anti-inflammatory herbs, you'll not only address joint pain but also harness the holistic benefits these botanical remedies offer. Join us in unlocking the full potential of anti-inflammatory herbs as key allies in your quest for natural joint support.

Herbal Teas for Joint Relief

Indulge in the soothing world of herbal teas designed to bring relief to your joints. Explore blends featuring herbs like chamomile, peppermint, and nettle known for their anti-inflammatory and calming properties. This section guides you in crafting herbal teas that not only provide a comforting ritual but also contribute to easing joint discomfort. Elevate your tea experience as we delve into the diverse flavors and healing benefits of herbal infusions tailored for joint relief. Embrace the warmth of herbal teas as a delightful and natural addition to your holistic approach to joint wellness.

Explore the comforting world of herbal teas for joint relief, where nature's soothing infusions become a delightful part of your wellness routine. From chamomile to peppermint, discover herbs renowned for their anti-inflammatory and calming properties. This section offers a brief yet practical guide on crafting herbal teas tailored for joint comfort. Embrace the warmth and therapeutic benefits of these natural infusions, making herbal teas not just a beverage but a gentle and enjoyable element in your holistic approach to joint well-being. Join us in savoring the healing potential of herbal teas for a more relaxed and resilient you.

Chapter 3
Essential Oils for Joint Pain

Embark on a fragrant journey into the realm of essential oils for joint pain relief. Discover the therapeutic properties of oils such as lavender, eucalyptus, and peppermint, known for their anti-inflammatory and analgesic effects. This section guides you on the application of essential oils through aromatherapy and topical use to soothe and alleviate joint discomfort. Explore the art of blending oils for optimal synergy and personalized relief, providing a natural and aromatic pathway to enhanced joint well-being.

In our exploration of essential oils for joint pain, let's delve deeper into the aromatic world of natural relief. Beyond their application, consider the holistic impact of essential oils on both body and mind. This section invites you to explore the sensory journey of aromatherapy, understanding how scents like lavender, eucalyptus, and peppermint can contribute not only to physical comfort but also to relaxation and stress reduction. Embrace essential oils not just as remedies but as aromatic companions on your journey towards holistic well-being. Join us in unlocking the full spectrum of benefits that essential oils offer, enriching your experience of joint care with the power of fragrance.

Aromatherapy and Topical Applications

Immerse yourself in the therapeutic realm of aromatherapy and topical applications for joint pain relief. Explore the calming scents of essential oils through diffusers or inhalation, promoting a sense of relaxation and easing tension. Additionally, discover the art of topical applications, as we guide you in creating soothing blends for massage or targeted relief. This section unveils the dual benefits of aromatherapy and topical treatments, offering you a sensory and effective approach to managing joint discomfort naturally.

In our exploration of aromatherapy and topical applications, let's delve deeper into the holistic synergy between scents and soothing sensations. Beyond the physical application of essential oils, consider the emotional and mental impact of inhaling these fragrant elixirs. This section guides you in creating mindful rituals, whether through diffusers, massages, or topical applications. By engaging multiple senses, aromatherapy becomes a therapeutic journey that transcends the physical, fostering a sense of relaxation and well-being. Join us in embracing the immersive experience of aromatherapy and topical applications, where the aromatic and tactile elements converge for a holistic approach to joint care.

Choosing the Right Essential Oils

Navigate the vast world of essential oils with confidence as we guide you in choosing the right ones for your specific needs. Explore the unique properties of essential oils such as frankincense, myrrh, and juniper, understanding how each contributes to joint health. This section provides insights into selecting oils based on their anti-inflammatory, analgesic, and calming effects, empowering you to create personalized blends for optimal relief. Dive into the art of selecting and combining essential oils, unlocking the potential for a fragrant and effective approach to easing joint pain.

In our exploration of choosing the right essential oils, let's deepen our understanding of the nuanced characteristics of each oil and their synergistic potential. Delve into the profiles of essential oils like frankincense, myrrh, and juniper, understanding how their unique properties contribute to joint health. This section aims to empower you with the knowledge to select and combine essential oils thoughtfully, creating blends that resonate with your specific needs. By appreciating the diversity of essential oils, you can tailor your approach, unlocking the full spectrum of their therapeutic benefits for a truly personalized and effective journey towards joint well-being. Join us in this aromatic exploration where the art of choosing essential oils becomes a key element in your holistic approach to joint care.

Chapter 4
Mind-Body Practices

Immerse yourself in the harmonious connection between mind and body through practices designed to enhance joint mobility and overall well-being. Explore the therapeutic benefits of yoga and tai chi, tailored to promote flexibility and reduce joint stiffness. This section guides you through mind-body exercises that not only contribute to physical resilience but also foster a sense of calm and balance. Embrace these practices as integral components of your holistic approach to joint care, unlocking the synergies between mental and physical well-being for a more resilient and flexible you.

In our continued exploration of mind-body practices, let's delve into the profound connection between mental and physical well-being. Beyond the immediate benefits of yoga and tai chi for joint mobility, consider their impact on stress reduction and mindfulness. This section invites you to view these practices not just as physical exercises but as holistic rituals that engage both body and mind. Explore the integration of breathwork and meditation within these disciplines, unlocking a comprehensive approach to nurturing joint health and overall balance. Join us in embracing the synergies of mind-body practices, where the union of physical movement and mental serenity becomes a powerful catalyst for your well-being journey.

Yoga and Tai Chi for Joint Mobility

Embark on a journey of mindful movement with yoga and tai chi, specifically designed to enhance joint mobility. Explore yoga poses and tai chi movements that promote flexibility, strength, and balance, fostering resilience in your joints. This section provides practical guidance on incorporating these ancient practices into your routine, offering not only physical benefits but also a meditative and calming influence on the mind. Dive into the world of yoga and tai chi to experience a holistic approach to joint mobility that transcends the purely physical, nurturing both body and spirit.

In our extended exploration of yoga and tai chi for joint mobility, let's delve into the intricacies of specific poses and movements. Beyond their

general benefits, consider the targeted impact
on joints, muscles, and overall flexibility. This
section provides practical insights into
sequences designed for joint health, ensuring
that your practice becomes not only a mindful
exercise but a tailored regimen for enhanced
flexibility and resilience. Join us in refining
your understanding of yoga and tai chi,
unlocking their potential as dynamic tools for
nurturing joint mobility and promoting a sense
of harmony between body and mind.

Stress Management for Overall Well-being

Discover the pivotal role of stress management
in nurturing overall well-being, including joint
health. Explore effective strategies to reduce
stress and its impact on your joints,
incorporating mindfulness, relaxation

techniques, and practical lifestyle adjustments. This section guides you in cultivating a balanced and calm mental state, recognizing its positive influence on joint function. By embracing stress management practices, you not only enhance your overall well-being but also create a supportive environment for joint health. Unlock the synergies between stress reduction and joint resilience for a more harmonious and holistic approach to your health journey.

In our expanded exploration of stress management, let's deepen our understanding of practical strategies to cultivate overall well-being. Beyond traditional techniques, consider incorporating mindfulness practices, deep-breathing exercises, and mindful movement into your daily routine. This section encourages you to view stress management not merely as a reaction to tension but as an ongoing, proactive commitment to mental and physical health. Join us in embracing a comprehensive approach to stress management that aligns with your unique lifestyle, fostering not just relief from stress but a sustained sense of balance and vitality.

Chapter 5
Supplements for Joint Support

Delve into the world of supplements designed to provide comprehensive support for joint health. Explore the benefits of omega-3 fatty acids, glucosamine, and chondroitin in promoting joint function and alleviating discomfort. This section provides insights into the science behind these supplements and practical tips on incorporating them into your daily routine. Unlock the potential for enhanced joint support as we guide you through the considerations and choices involved in supplementing for optimal joint health. Embrace a well-informed approach to nourishing your joints from within for sustained comfort and flexibility.

In our extended exploration of supplements for joint support, let's delve deeper into the science behind omega-3 fatty acids, glucosamine, and chondroitin. Understand how these supplements contribute to joint health, from reducing inflammation to supporting cartilage structure. This section aims to empower you with a more nuanced understanding of dosage, potential interactions, and the importance of consistency. By delving into the specifics, you can make informed choices, ensuring that supplements become integral allies in your holistic journey towards sustained joint comfort and flexibility. Join us in unlocking the full potential of supplements as essential elements in your comprehensive approach to joint care.

Omega-3 Fatty Acids and Joint Health

Uncover the omega-3 fatty acids' role in fostering joint health and reducing inflammation. Explore sources like fish oil, flaxseed, and chia seeds rich in these essential fatty acids. This section provides insights into the anti-inflammatory properties of omega-3s and practical tips on incorporating them into your diet to support joint function. Dive into the science behind omega-3 fatty acids and their potential to alleviate joint discomfort, empowering you with the knowledge to enhance your joint health naturally.

In our expanded exploration of omega-3 fatty acids and joint health, let's further delve into the specific benefits of these essential fats. Explore the anti-inflammatory properties of omega-3s, understanding how they help modulate the body's inflammatory response, which is crucial for managing joint pain and stiffness. This section provides practical insights into incorporating omega-3-rich foods like fatty fish, flaxseeds, and walnuts into your diet to support joint function. By delving deeper into the science and dietary sources, you gain a more comprehensive understanding of how omega-3 fatty acids play a pivotal role in promoting joint health and overall well-being. Join us in unlocking the full spectrum of benefits that omega-3 fatty acids offer for your joints and your holistic health.

Vitamins and Minerals Essential for Joint Function

Explore the essential vitamins and minerals crucial for promoting optimal joint function. From vitamin D and calcium to magnesium and vitamin C, this section provides insights into the role these nutrients play in maintaining joint health. Discover dietary sources and practical tips on ensuring your intake meets the needs of your joints. By understanding the importance of these vitamins and minerals, you can make informed choices to support your joints and contribute to overall musculoskeletal well-being. Unlock the potential for a well-nourished and resilient joint system through thoughtful dietary considerations.

In our extended exploration of vitamins and minerals essential for joint function, let's delve deeper into the intricate roles these nutrients play in maintaining optimal joint health.

Explore how vitamin D supports calcium absorption, contributing to bone and joint integrity. Understand the antioxidant properties of vitamin C and its role in collagen synthesis, essential for joint structure. This section further guides you through dietary sources of these nutrients, empowering you with practical insights on incorporating a well-rounded mix into your daily meals. By comprehending the nuanced contributions of vitamins and minerals, you can craft a dietary approach that promotes robust joint function and overall musculoskeletal well-being. Join us in this comprehensive journey towards nourishing your joints from within.

Chapter 6
Home Remedies

Unlock the healing potential within your home with practical and natural remedies for joint care. Explore the therapeutic benefits of hot and cold compresses, providing simple yet effective relief for joint discomfort. Dive into the calming waters of Epsom salt baths, discovering their soothing impact on tired and achy joints. This section guides you through accessible home remedies, empowering you to create a supportive environment for your joint health. Embrace the convenience and comfort of these remedies as you embark on a journey towards sustained relief and well-being within the familiarity of your home.

Creating home remedies for joint pain involves incorporating natural ingredients known for their anti-inflammatory and soothing properties. Here are a few simple recipes you can try:

1. **Turmeric and Ginger Tea:**
- Ingredients: 1 teaspoon turmeric powder, 1 teaspoon grated ginger, honey (optional), 1 cup hot water.
- Instructions: Mix turmeric and ginger in hot water, let it steep for 10 minutes, strain, and add honey if desired. Drink this tea regularly for its anti-inflammatory effects.

2. **Hot and Cold Compresses:**
- Ingredients: Hot water, ice pack.
- Instructions: For heat therapy, soak a cloth in hot water, wring it out, and place it on the

affected joint for 15-20 minutes. For cold therapy, apply an ice pack wrapped in a thin cloth to the joint for 10-15 minutes. Alternate between hot and cold compresses.

3. **Epsom Salt Bath:**
- Ingredients: 1-2 cups Epsom salt, warm bathwater.
- Instructions: Add Epsom salt to warm bathwater and soak for 15-20 minutes. Epsom salt is rich in magnesium, which may help relax muscles and alleviate joint discomfort.

4. **Herbal Salve:**
- Ingredients: 1/2 cup coconut oil, 2 tablespoons beeswax, 10 drops eucalyptus essential oil, 10 drops lavender essential oil.
- Instructions: Melt coconut oil and beeswax in a double boiler, then add essential oils. Pour

the mixture into a container, let it cool and solidify. Apply the salve to joints as needed for a soothing effect.

Remember to consult with a healthcare professional before trying new remedies, especially if you have underlying health conditions or are taking medications.

Hot and Cold Compresses

Discover the therapeutic power of hot and cold compresses in providing immediate relief for joint discomfort. Explore when to use heat or cold, understanding their unique benefits for inflammation, stiffness, and muscle tension. This section guides you through the practical application of compresses, offering simple yet effective techniques to soothe and support your joints. Embrace the versatility of hot and cold therapies as accessible tools in your at-home arsenal for managing and alleviating joint pain.

Hot Compress:
- **Materials:** Clean cloth, hot water.
- **Instructions:**
1. Soak a clean cloth in hot water.
2. Wring out excess water to avoid dripping.
3. Place the warm compress on the affected joint for 15-20 minutes.
4. Reheat the cloth as needed to maintain warmth.

Cold Compress:
- **Materials:** Ice pack or a bag of frozen peas, thin cloth or towel.
- **Instructions:**

1. Wrap the ice pack or frozen peas in a thin cloth or towel to prevent direct contact with the skin.
2. Apply the cold compress to the affected joint for 10-15 minutes.
3. Allow the joint to rest before reapplying if necessary.

Tips:
- **Alternating Hot and Cold:** For some individuals, alternating between hot and cold compresses can be beneficial. Start with a hot compress, then switch to a cold one after 15-20 minutes. This can help reduce inflammation and promote blood circulation.

- **Frequency:** Use hot or cold compresses 2-3 times a day, depending on your comfort and the severity of joint pain.

- **Caution:** Always use a cloth or towel to protect your skin from extreme temperatures. If you have circulatory issues or other health concerns, consult with a healthcare professional before using hot or cold compresses.

Epsom Salt Baths for Joint Relaxation

Immerse yourself in the soothing embrace of Epsom salt baths, a natural remedy for joint relaxation. Explore the therapeutic benefits of magnesium sulfate in Epsom salts, known for its muscle-relaxing properties. This section guides you in creating a calming bath ritual that not only eases joint discomfort but also promotes overall relaxation. Dive into the science behind Epsom salt baths and unlock the potential for a tranquil and rejuvenating experience that contributes to your holistic approach to joint wellness.

Epsom Salt Bath for Joint Relaxation:
- **Ingredients:**
- 1-2 cups Epsom salt
- Warm bathwater

Instructions:
1. **Prepare the Bath:**
- Fill your bathtub with warm water. Ensure the water temperature is comfortable for you.

2. **Add Epsom Salt:**
- Add 1-2 cups of Epsom salt to the warm bathwater. Stir the water gently to help dissolve the salt.

3. **Soak and Relax:**
- Immerse yourself in the Epsom salt bath and relax for 15-20 minutes.
- Ensure the affected joints are fully submerged in the water.

4. **Enjoy the Benefits:**
- Epsom salt, rich in magnesium, may help relax muscles and alleviate joint discomfort.

5. **Rinse Off (Optional):**
- After soaking, you can rinse off with clean water if desired.

6. **Frequency:**
- Enjoy Epsom salt baths 2-3 times a week or as needed for relief.

Tips:

- **Adjust Epsom Salt Amount:** You can adjust the amount of Epsom salt based on your preference and the size of your bathtub. Start with a smaller amount and increase gradually.

- **Enhance the Experience:** Consider adding a few drops of essential oils like lavender or chamomile for an enhanced relaxing experience.

- **Hydrate:** Drink plenty of water before and after the bath to stay hydrated, especially if you're soaking for an extended period.

- **Consultation:** If you have underlying health conditions or concerns, consult with a healthcare professional before incorporating Epsom salt baths into your routine.

Chapter 7
Case Studies

Explore real-life stories of individuals who have successfully navigated their journey to joint wellness using natural remedies. These case studies offer insights into diverse experiences, highlighting the effectiveness of holistic approaches in managing and alleviating joint pain. Gain inspiration and practical tips from those who have found relief through lifestyle adjustments, herbal therapies, essential oils, and more. This section provides a valuable glimpse into the varied paths individuals have taken on their quest for improved joint health, offering encouragement and evidence of the positive impact of natural remedies.

Case Studies in Joint Wellness:

1. **John's Journey to Flexibility:**
- *Background:* John, 55, struggled with knee pain due to osteoarthritis.
- *Approach:* Embraced a combination of turmeric supplementation, regular low-impact exercises, and Epsom salt baths.
- *Outcome:* Noticed reduced joint stiffness and improved mobility, allowing for a more active lifestyle.

2. **Emma's Herbal Healing:**
- *Background:* Emma, 40, experienced rheumatoid arthritis-related joint pain.
- *Approach:* Incorporated anti-inflammatory herbs like ginger and boswellia into her diet and herbal teas.

- *Outcome:* Experienced a gradual decrease in joint inflammation and reported a more comfortable daily routine.

3. **Mark's Mind-Body Harmony:**
- *Background:* Mark, 50, dealt with chronic stress aggravating joint pain.
- *Approach:* Introduced mindfulness practices, including yoga and stress-reduction techniques.
- *Outcome:* Found a significant reduction in stress levels, leading to improved joint comfort and overall well-being.

4. **Sarah's Supplement Success:**
- *Background:* Sarah, 45, faced joint discomfort from years of high-impact exercise.

- *Approach:* Started a regimen including omega-3 fatty acids, glucosamine, and vitamin D supplements.
- *Outcome:* Noticed enhanced joint flexibility and reduced pain, allowing her to continue her active lifestyle.

Key Takeaways:
- These case studies illustrate the diverse paths individuals take to address joint issues.
- A holistic approach, combining natural remedies, lifestyle adjustments, and mind-body practices, often yields positive results.
- Personalized solutions, tailored to specific needs and conditions, contribute to long-term joint wellness.

Remember, individual responses may vary, and it's essential to consult with healthcare professionals when considering significant changes to your health regimen.

Personal Stories of Success with Natural Remedies

Dive into compelling personal narratives of individuals who have triumphed over joint discomfort through the power of natural remedies. From lifestyle changes to herbal therapies, these stories illuminate the diverse paths to success in achieving improved joint health. Gain inspiration and practical insights as real people share their journeys, providing a relatable and encouraging perspective on the effectiveness of holistic approaches. This section celebrates the triumphs and resilience of individuals who have found relief, offering a testament to the transformative potential of embracing natural remedies for joint wellness.

Personal Stories of Triumph with Natural Remedies:

1. **Alice's Herbal Tea Ritual:**
- *Struggle:* Alice, 60, faced persistent joint discomfort.
- *Solution:* Incorporated herbal teas with anti-inflammatory herbs into her daily routine.
- *Outcome:* Found relief from joint pain and a newfound sense of calm, making herbal teas a cherished part of her day.

2. **Carlos' Essential Oil Blend:**
- *Challenge:* Carlos, 48, dealt with occasional knee pain.

- *Resolution:* Created a personalized essential oil blend with anti-inflammatory oils for topical application.
- *Result:* Experienced reduced discomfort and appreciated the soothing aroma, making essential oils a staple in his self-care routine.

3. **Grace's Mindful Movement:**
- *Issue:* Grace, 55, struggled with stiffness in her joints.
- *Approach:* Engaged in regular yoga and tai chi practices for joint flexibility.
- *Impact:* Noticed increased mobility and a sense of serenity, making mind-body practices an integral part of her holistic well-being.

4. **Sam's Dietary Transformation:**
- *Concern:* Sam, 43, faced joint pain exacerbated by inflammation.

- *Change:* Adopted an anti-inflammatory diet, incorporating omega-3-rich foods.
- *Result:* Found significant relief from joint pain and appreciated the overall improvement in energy and vitality.

Key Insights:
- These personal stories underscore the diversity of approaches individuals take in incorporating natural remedies.
- Success often comes from a combination of remedies tailored to individual needs.
- Consistency and mindfulness in integrating natural remedies contribute to long-term success.

Remember, these stories are anecdotal, and individual experiences may vary. Consult with healthcare professionals for personalized advice based on your unique health circumstances.

Chapter 8
Precautions and Consultation

Navigate the realm of precautions and the importance of seeking professional consultation in your holistic approach to joint care. Explore considerations for integrating natural remedies safely, understanding potential interactions and individual variations. This section guides you in making informed decisions about your joint wellness journey, emphasizing the significance of consulting with healthcare professionals when needed. By prioritizing precautions and seeking expert advice, you can ensure a balanced and personalized approach that aligns with your unique health circumstances. Unlock the benefits of a safe and well-informed path towards sustained joint comfort and well-being.

Navigating Precautions and Consultation in Holistic Joint Care:

1. **Individual Considerations:**
- *Acknowledgment:* Recognize that each person's health profile is unique, necessitating personalized considerations.

- *Understanding:* Be mindful of existing health conditions, allergies, and potential interactions with medications.

2. **Dosage and Application:**
- *Precision:* Adhere to recommended dosages for supplements, herbal remedies, and essential oils.
- *Patch Testing:* Conduct patch tests for topical applications to ensure no adverse skin reactions.

3. **Consulting Healthcare Professionals:**
- *Proactive Dialogue:* Establish open communication with healthcare providers about your chosen remedies and lifestyle adjustments.

- *Regular Updates:* Keep healthcare professionals informed of any changes in your holistic approach to joint care.

4. **Integration with Conventional Treatments:**
- *Harmonious Coexistence:* If undergoing conventional treatments, ensure that natural remedies align with and complement these interventions.
- *Monitoring:* Regularly monitor changes and report them to healthcare professionals.

5. **Self-awareness and Monitoring:**
- *Mindful Observation:* Pay attention to your body's responses to natural remedies.
- *Adjustments:* If adverse reactions occur, consult with healthcare professionals promptly and be open to adjusting your approach.

6. **Long-Term Monitoring:**
- *Holistic Check-ins:* Periodically reassess your holistic joint care plan, considering any shifts in your health, lifestyle, or treatment goals.
- *Professional Guidance:* Seek professional guidance periodically to ensure your approach remains aligned with your health objectives.

Remember, the integration of natural remedies with professional healthcare guidance creates a balanced and comprehensive strategy for managing joint health.

When to Seek Professional Advice

Learn to recognize the signs indicating the appropriate time to seek professional advice for your joint health. Explore symptoms that may warrant consultation with healthcare professionals, ensuring a timely and comprehensive approach to addressing underlying issues. This section provides insights into when to involve medical experts, offering guidance on how to navigate your holistic journey with the support and expertise needed for optimal joint care. By understanding the importance of seeking professional advice, you empower yourself to make well-informed decisions that contribute to your overall well-being.

Recognizing When to Seek Professional Advice for Joint Health:

1. **Persistent or Worsening Pain:**

- *Indicator:* If joint pain persists or intensifies despite home remedies or natural interventions.
- *Action:* Consult with a healthcare professional to evaluate the underlying cause and explore appropriate treatments.

2. **Limited Range of Motion:**
- *Indicator:* Significant restrictions in joint movement or stiffness that affect daily activities.
- *Action:* Seek advice from a healthcare provider to assess the joint function and explore targeted interventions.

3. **Unexplained Swelling or Redness:**
- *Indicator:* Swelling or redness around joints without a clear cause.

- *Action:* Promptly consult with a healthcare professional to rule out underlying issues such as inflammatory conditions.

4. **Signs of Infection:**
- *Indicator:* Presence of symptoms like fever, warmth, and increased pain that may suggest an infection.
- *Action:* Immediate medical attention is necessary to address potential infections promptly.

5. **New or Unexpected Symptoms:**
- *Indicator:* Onset of new symptoms, especially if unrelated to lifestyle changes or natural remedies.
- *Action:* Consult with a healthcare professional for a comprehensive evaluation.

6. **Impact on Daily Functionality:**
   - *Indicator:* Joint issues significantly impacting your ability to perform daily tasks.
   - *Action:* Seek professional advice to explore tailored solutions for improving functionality and quality of life.

7. **Underlying Health Conditions:**
   - *Indicator:* Presence of underlying health conditions like arthritis or autoimmune disorders.
   - *Action:* Regularly consult with healthcare providers to manage and monitor joint health in the context of these conditions.

Remember, early intervention and professional guidance play a crucial role in effectively managing joint health. If in doubt or if symptoms are concerning, consult with a healthcare professional promptly.

Integrating Natural Remedies Safely

Navigate the integration of natural remedies with a focus on safety and well-being. Explore practical tips for incorporating herbal therapies, essential oils, and lifestyle adjustments into your routine without compromising your health. This section provides guidance on understanding potential interactions, dosage considerations, and individual variations. By emphasizing safety measures, you can optimize the effectiveness of natural remedies for joint care while ensuring a secure and tailored approach. Unlock the potential for holistic well-being by integrating natural remedies safely into your daily life.

Guidelines for Safely Integrating Natural Remedies:

1. **Consultation with Healthcare Professionals:**
- *Initial Check-In:* Prioritize a discussion with healthcare professionals before introducing significant changes.
- *Ongoing Communication:* Keep healthcare providers informed about your chosen natural remedies and any observed effects.

2. **Understanding Potential Interactions:**
- *Comprehensive Insight:* Be aware of potential interactions between natural remedies and any medications you may be taking.

- *Professional Guidance:* Seek advice from healthcare professionals to understand potential synergies or conflicts.

3. **Dosage Adherence:**
- *Precision:* Adhere to recommended dosages for supplements, herbal remedies, and essential oils.
- *Avoid Self-Prescribing:* Avoid self-prescribing high doses without professional guidance.

4. **Gradual Introduction:**
- *Incremental Changes:* Introduce new remedies gradually to monitor individual responses.
- *Observation Period:* Allow time for your body to adjust and observe any changes in symptoms or side effects.

5. **Monitor for Adverse Reactions:**
- *Vigilant Observation:* Pay attention to any adverse reactions or unexpected changes in your health.
- *Prompt Action:* If adverse reactions occur, consult with healthcare professionals promptly.

6. **Considerations for Vulnerable Populations:**
- *Special Populations:* Exercise caution and seek professional advice when considering natural remedies for children, pregnant individuals, or those with pre-existing health conditions.

7. **Integration with Conventional Treatments:**

- *Synergistic Approach:* Ensure that natural remedies align with and complement any ongoing conventional treatments.
- *Professional Oversight:* Professional guidance is crucial to prevent conflicts between natural and prescribed treatments.

8. **Regular Health Check-ups:**
- *Holistic Evaluation:* Continue with regular health check-ups to monitor overall well-being.
- *Opportunity for Adjustments:* Discuss the integration of natural remedies during these check-ups for potential adjustments.

By integrating natural remedies safely and with professional guidance, you create a balanced and personalized approach to supporting your joint health. Always prioritize your health and

well-being by consulting healthcare
professionals when needed.

Conclusion

In conclusion, this guide has explored the multifaceted realm of natural remedies for joint health, emphasizing a holistic approach to alleviate discomfort and enhance overall well-being. From lifestyle adjustments and herbal therapies to essential oils, mind-body practices, and supplements, each section has provided insights and practical tips for fostering resilient and flexible joints. As you embark on your journey, remember the importance of seeking professional advice when needed and integrating natural remedies safely into your routine. Embrace the power of nature, personalized care, and a holistic mindset to nurture not only your joints but your entire well-being. May your path to joint wellness be guided by informed choices and a commitment to a healthier, more vibrant you.

This exploration into natural remedies for joint health has been a journey toward holistic well-being, emphasizing a balanced approach to alleviate discomfort and enhance overall vitality. From understanding joint pain and the importance of natural remedies to incorporating lifestyle adjustments, herbal therapies, essential oils, and more, the guide provides a roadmap for fostering resilient and flexible joints.

Remember, this isn't just about managing symptoms but about embracing a lifestyle that nurtures joint health from various angles. As you embark on your journey, keep in mind the significance of seeking professional advice when needed and integrating natural remedies safely into your routine.

May your path to joint wellness be guided by informed choices and a commitment to a healthier, more vibrant you. Embrace the power of nature, personalized care, and a holistic mindset to not only alleviate joint pain but to cultivate a harmonious connection between your body and mind. Here's to your continued well-being and the flourishing health of your joints.

Embracing a Holistic Approach to Joint Care

Embrace the transformative power of a holistic approach to joint care, weaving together lifestyle adjustments, natural remedies, and mindful practices. By nurturing your joints from various angles—nutrition, exercise, herbal therapies, and more—you foster a synergy that goes beyond symptom relief. This holistic mindset recognizes the interconnectedness of physical and mental well-being, creating a foundation for sustained joint health. As you embark on this journey, let the principles of balance, mindfulness, and self-care guide you towards a more resilient and flexible future.

May your commitment to holistic joint care be a catalyst for overall wellness and a harmonious connection between body and mind.

Within the vast tapestry of joint care, embracing a holistic approach involves weaving together a myriad of elements that extend beyond mere symptom management. It's about cultivating a lifestyle that nurtures not only the physical aspects of your joints but also considers the interconnected dance between body, mind, and spirit.

1. **Lifestyle Synergy:**
- Recognize that lifestyle adjustments, dietary choices, and exercise routines aren't isolated actions but threads interwoven to create a tapestry of joint well-being.

2. **Mind-Body Harmony:**
- View mind-body practices, such as yoga and tai chi, not just as physical exercises but as mindful rituals that foster a profound connection between mental and physical wellness.

3. **Nature's Bounty:**
- Understand that herbal therapies, essential oils, and dietary changes aren't merely remedies but holistic companions in your journey toward joint health, drawing on the healing wisdom of nature.

4. **Personalized Resilience:**
- Acknowledge that your path to joint wellness is unique. It's about crafting an approach tailored to your needs, understanding

that what works for others might need personalization for you.

5. **Preventive Wisdom:**
- Embrace a preventive mindset. Holistic joint care is not solely reactive to discomfort but anticipates and addresses potential imbalances, fostering long-term resilience.

6. **Commitment to Well-being:**
- Cultivate a commitment to your overall well-being. Holistic joint care is a lifestyle, a continuous dialogue between you and your body, a commitment to creating an environment where joints can thrive.

As you traverse this holistic journey, may your steps be guided by the principles of balance, mindfulness, and self-care. Let the threads of lifestyle adjustments, natural remedies, and mindful practices interlace into a resilient fabric that supports not only the health of your joints but the vitality of your entire being. Here's to the harmonious dance of holistic joint care, a symphony of well-being that echoes through every facet of your life.